HEALTHY?
SAYS WHO?

HEALTHY? SAYS WHO?

THE MOST CONTROVERSIAL BOOK YOU WILL EVER READ

DR. GEORGE F. NARYSHKIN

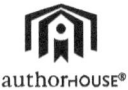

authorHOUSE®

AuthorHouse™ LLC
1663 Liberty Drive
Bloomington, IN 47403
www.authorhouse.com
Phone: 1-800-839-8640

Published by AuthorHouse   02/10/2014

ISBN: 978-1-4918-5289-7 (sc)
ISBN: 978-1-4918-5287-3 (hc)
ISBN: 978-1-4918-5288-0 (e)

Library of Congress Control Number: 2014901077

Contents

Chapter Eight

Chapter Nine

Dedicated to

My 2 children, Ana-Maria and Nikolas Ryan
So that they might not suffer from the
problems discussed in this book

And

My mother and father who raised and nurtured
me in an environment which promoted curiosity
in nature and permitted me to explore it

And

My wife Nazilma who put up with me while
I ranted about the topics in this book

And

The Ghosts of Temple University
Dental School of the 1980s

Title—by Bill Kaba

Prologue

Who am I?

Hello. My name is Dr. George F. Naryshkin. I have been a practicing dentist for 30 years now. I will tell you of my background as I feel it is necessary for you to both understand my points of view and for you to understand this book.

I attended Toms River High School North in Toms River NJ. My favorite activities were the band and track and field. I played trombone, and then tuba in the marching and stage bands and enjoyed them very much. I pole vaulted on the track team and this required not only physical training, but a lot of mental strength. I had to be certain of my abilities.

I attended Rutgers College of Rutgers University before obtaining a sudden love of geology and transferring to Baylor University where I studied geology and completed my senior thesis in the topic of vertebrate paleontology.

The study of geology gave me the experience of and understanding of the importance of defining a problem (knowing what question to ask) and then defining my intentions in solving the problem, and of how I would go about obtaining data and presenting that data, not an agenda.

My instructors, most notably Dr. O.T. Hayward, emphasized the importance of accurate collections of data, and the presentation of all data, even if it disproved your theory. Data was of most importance as was the correct presentation of your results.

I attended USAF pilot training at Reese AFB in Lubbock, Texas and received my pilot's wings there. Military pilot training was very challenging and taught all pilots the importance of knowing all items instructed to them. Most written exams required a %100 in order to graduate and to continue in your assigned aircraft. There was no room for interpretation. 200 knots on touch down was 200 knots. It wasn't up to what your friend did or said. I enjoyed the Air Force mostly because of this black/white thinking. And it did not matter if it hurt your feelings to know the truth. If an item was important, the instructors let you know that. And 3 major goofs and you were released from training with no chance of returning, ever.

Military pilot training taught me that there are absolute limits such as a maximum airspeed an aircraft could be flown at, and that the limit was not open to interpretation or belief. What the data showed was what we followed, no discussion.

I attended dental school at Temple University in 1982. Temple had either a culture or requirement that all instructors or professors had military experience.

This gave me more benefits than I realized at the time. Most professors had retired from the military and so had some security, i.e. they did not have to be politically correct or "nice" to people in fear of needing a future job at a dental office. Because of this they spoke the truth (the truth being what the data showed) and they faced incorrect thinking individuals head on (professors or students). Of course there were some incompetent instructors who simply took up space, but the majority fit the mould of truth tellers.

I did not realize what this would mean to me until perhaps 10-20 years later when my professors seemed to reincarnate themselves in me. As I came across dentists or physicians who were telling me or patients strange things, I could hear the voices of the past in my head and I began to imitate them in their honor and in doing what was correct.

I consider one of my main strengths to be my ability to see the big picture. By that I mean, for example, that to grow tomatoes one does not have to understand biochemistry or agriculture. I just know that if I place a seed in soil and add water, a tomato plant will grow. That is the big picture. No need to get lost in the details of biochemistry unless you want to analyze a specific problem.

A few themes that my professors tattooed into my brain were 1. That the world was getting dumber. The average person, and even science majors no longer knew what science was. They could not and did not discern between an article in People Magazine and a peer reviewed scientific journal. Dentists were practicing on patients using methods told to them by sales persons rather than their professors in school.

Speakers were openly ridiculed in front of students when they presented instruction using unscientific evidence.

I will give more specifics later in this book.

I have also been a patient (both dental and medical) and have experiences to learn from.

Although now I work as a general dentist performing mostly oral surgical procedures on patients, I consider myself to be a naturalist who enjoys studying all aspects of life.

My family

My family includes an ob/gyn (father), pathologist(sister), dentist (brother) and current and past relatives who were physicians as well. As a result I had great access to medical and dental periodicals and points of view.

I have reached that time in my life where I am free as my professors were, in that I do not have to muffle my opinion. I do not have to be politically correct for fear of insulting a future employer or patient. I am now free to tell the truth and to "stick it in their faces" so to speak.

Disclaimer

I have included this disclaimer in order to hopefully avoid being contacted by the medically illiterate.

This book is meant as entertainment. I approach failed medical and dental treatment by making professionals and laymen alike, aware that our professionals have adopted the practice of consensus rather than science in diagnosing and treating patients.

I do not wish to be contacted by a physician who asks me if I can recite all pathogens in the world. I cannot.

I do not want to hear from a dentist who says "but most dentists do this, or that". I do not care was the consensus is. If I am the only dentist who treats a patient according to data and science, then I am correct and am providing a great service to my patient. I will not refuse treat a patient out of fear of going to court over a complaint, and the other side's attorney pays someone to say he is an expert and that he disagrees with me. I don't care.

You will only attempt to argue with me if you are one of the unenlightened, and I have no time for a physician who will argue that there is plenty of evidence (meaning plenty of physicians who agree with him) to back up his actions when there is none.

It is with my ability to stand up to consensus of the ignorant that I write this book in order to enlighten you of the problems with society and physicians and dentists which causes many to follow the crowd while receiving no medical or dental benefit.

Chapter One

What is my purpose?

The reason why I wrote this book is to vent steam at my frustration of what has happened to sound science and reason, and to attempt to point my finger, not at individuals or even scientific communities, but at our entire society and the politics of cause.

I am a libertarian and conservative, but I will attempt to not lecture and not discuss politics. I also use simple terms as I am a simple man and look at the world in simple ways.

I want people to know the truth of why they go to the doctor and the truth of the diagnosis or treatments they decide to have performed on their unique bodies of which they will only have one. The truth means data, not what people say.

This book was published for its entertainment value and is aimed at both professionals and the general public. I know I will have many enemies after this books' publication, but so be it. It is exactly because of the fear of creating enemies that the problems I present in this book exist.

Although all facts or studies I sight in this book are real and true, I cannot site many references as I have long ago, cleaned out my office and had to get rid of hundreds of journals and articles. So I cannot refer to this work as a scientific one. But I know what I know, and I know what I don't know. I know what data does exist. If you choose to live by my writings, you will have to research the subject and come up with your own conclusions.

I did not address every topic of medicine or dentistry as that was not my goal. This is not a self help book or a book on alternative medicine. I only chose to discuss topics in which I found doctors or dentists in the wrong based on what data tells us and what we were taught in dental school or medical school and which was data based.

I observed that it is part of our culture for most persons to think that they cannot live a normal life unless they follow the insurance company line of going to the doctor and dentist every 6 months. I see this as only causing stress on a person and in lessening their ability to enjoy their short life.

I am not unsympathetic to those who do have illness such as cancer or other diseases. I just want to present facts as I have observed in correctly performed research so that you can decide if you want to participate in bad medical practices.

I write this book in the hopes of setting everyone free from this insane ritual.

Just What is my Beef?

My beef is in what has happened with medicine and dentistry in this country, and that I am very disappointed in my colleagues. There exist many basic principles we were all taught (I am sure) in our medical and dental schools. My instructors emphasized that they were witnessing a decline in the understanding of what science was, even to those who graduated science schools such as medical and dental schools. I have noticed this in graduates of earth sciences schools as well.

Medical professionals are abandoning safety measures and tried and true procedures as well as abandoning data.

Courses were given on how to distinguish between a pop-culture article and a peer reviewed scientific article, in an ill fated attempt to make graduates more intelligent.

If all that mattered was that scientists were not so intelligent, what would be so bad about that? The problem is that doctors/dentists are supposed to be the leaders in medical information to their patients. There is enough garbage floating around about science and our bodies. The leaders are there to hush ignorance and at lease lessen the misinformation. Instead I see the doctors/dentists causing and perpetuating misinformation.

It is true that all practitioners, including me, practice superstition. By that I mean that if we get a good result, either financially, or professionally (we cure the patient), we will continue to perform the same procedure or to prescribe the same medication. I am not criticizing this, as long as it does not violate patient safety.

And this matters because why? Because there are 2 types of people in this world when it comes to our bodies. The first one feels safe if they follow what they hear on t.v. or read in a people magazine. They will only feel safe if they have every test performed on them that they can find in their health insurance manual.

The other type of person wants to enjoy their life and only fix something that's broken. They do not want to sit and use their free time to ponder of what might kill them.

Also, most of my arguments either while practicing dentistry or being examined by physicians, were about misinformation. Either my patients wanted to know why I was not treating them as another dentist was, or my physician could not understand why I would question a diagnosis or treatment recommendation. I was fighting misinformation and the patients and physicians resisted because I was insulting their beliefs. Logic could not reach them.

I do not want anyone to take my word for what I have claimed to be data in this book. I expect you to investigate on your own each topic and then decide for yourself. The only problem is that most of you will not be able to see thru all the propaganda on the internet which is slanted towards convincing people that they <u>need</u> "health care", and that only the government can get this for you, and only they can know what you need.

Almost all "health" advice you see on tv or hear from friends is driven by political agenda, not sound scientific data.

Chapter Two

What you need to know

In order for you to understand the points I will be making in this book, I have decided to start you off with some definitions.

Health (medical usage)—If something increases your health it causes an organism to live longer than the average age of its population and to have less major illnesses such as cancers or diabetes. There is no "healthy" diet as far as medicine is concerned.

Health (pop-culture usage) means you have a sense of well being. It is a political word as socialists use this word to describe what they want you to buy or consume. A "healthy" diet has no scientific meaning. If it does mean something, how is it measured? It simply means "I want you to eat this and don't ask why". Also, if you are injured, it does not mean you are not "healthy" medically speaking. It means you are not "fit"(see below).

The term "health" was first incorrectly used in American pop-culture sometime in the 70's when the NFL (national football league) began using it to describe an injury free situation. Fit would have been the appropriate term to use. But the media ran with it and it eventually made it's way into medical insurance which became "health" insurances.

And currently the media uses the word health to mean either fit or medical health and this is further driving ignorance in our country.

Anyone selling anything will add at the end of the advertisement "and it is healthy too". They know no one will question this. No one asks "what do you mean by healthy"? or "show me the data".

Fit (physically fit)—This means you can function to a level you desire. It has nothing to do with how long you live or what illness you make contract. Most people will be or feel more fit if they eat less and exercise more. This has nothing to do with health (medical usage). More on this later.

Standard of care—has no medical usage. It is a phrase lawyers use to convince a jury that they are correct and not the other side. There is no reference for the standard of care. When an individual uses it when speaking to a patient, for example, he wants the patient to think that he is really smart and that the prescribed treatment is a good one. In fact it means nothing except that you are being taken advantage of.

Scientific method—method by which people gain knowledge when investigating phenomena. This must be based on empirical and measurable evidence based on scientific reasoning. Simply put, the person claiming to have scientific evidence must define his investigation and demonstrate his techniques for gathering his data. All must use good reasoning.

An example of a non-scientific conclusion versus a scientifically backed up conclusion is that of Vitamin C. For decades, citizens as well as physicians have promoted the use of vitamin c to prevent the common cold. There was never any evidence that this was a justified practice. In the 1970s an institute was started in the UK called the "Cold Institute", whose purpose was to study the common cold under scientific controls and procedures. Volunteers agreed to be sequestered in rooms where temperature and possible infectious viruses and bacteria could be controlled. Patients were exposed to the virus causing the common cold and then were isolated from other patients and they were given vitamin c. Others were not given the vitamin c. I do not recall how many patients were involved in each study, but it was statistically significant that the vitamin c had no effect on preventing or treating the common cold.

Any stories about a person taking vitamin c and having a cold go away, were simply anecdotal, meaning it was not obtained using the scientific method under controlled conditions.

In order that a study of the benefit of taking a daily vitamin be considered to be valid, parameters must be set, and the variables must be controlled and isolated.

Asking a person if he took a vitamin once a day for his entire life is not scientific. He must be observed to have taken his vitamin and the scientist must provide the vitamin so its contents are known. And the control group (a group of humans who do not take a vitamin) must be observed to be sure they have not consumed something that contains vitamins.

Even something as simple as the above is not understood by many students who graduated medical or dental school.

Scientific (pop-culture)—anything someone hears another person say is scientific. It has no place in true understanding of scientific phenomenon.

Superstition—Most physicians and dentists practice by this. A dentist uses a certain adhesive for a restoration (filling) and the filling does not fall out for years. He then attributes this success to the brand of adhesive when it may have nothing to do with it, but he continues to only use that brand. It is based on belief and many times it is a good thing. It does not, however indicate that it is correct or has a basis in science.

What is really scientific? How can I know this?

Examples of statements that are not scientific (have no measurable evidence)

1. Radiation causes cancer—Only government sponsored papers claim to have evidence which concludes radiation causes cancer. I was not taught that radiation causes cancer in dental school and although I have searched long and hard, I have not found independent studies which demonstrate radiation causes cancer. I have found evidence in independent studies which shows that radiation exposure prevents cancer.

2. Blood pressure matters—again, I have not found any scientific evidence to support this statement. All I hear are things people say. And that is not science. Blood pressure is a symptom, not a disease. The numbers a doctor tells you that you must be below have no meaning. They are arbitrary. Independent studies demonstrate that if a doctor alters your blood pressure reading to

below 150/90, it does not benefit anyone except the doctor as he can smile inside knowing he "did something"! It is something that can be measured (the reading) so he can claim victory. Evidence shows that a person does not live longer if their blood pressure is lowered. There is evidence to show that if after a stroke, if a patient's blood pressure is lowered, they are more likely to have a serious stroke.

3. Institutionalized study—There are studies which can be defined as "independent research" and "institutionalized research". We were taught in dental school that no one has ever conceived cancer as a result of exposure to radiation, but we were also taught that the "institutionalized" view of the matter is that there was. So led aprons are NOT required for the dentist to use on a patient when exposing them to radiation, but institutions want them to. Institutions are given money by politicians, and politicians want their voters to think they are keeping them safe. So the institutionalized studies are doctored to fit an agenda.

Chapter Three

Just What is Healthy?

Medical Myths

Going to the doctor for regular check-ups makes you live longer

Blood pressure matters

There is a healthy diet that benefits you

Going for regular breast, prostate and cervical exams makes you live longer

Radiation causes cancer

Everyone must find out if they have anything, any condition that can be named.

As stated above in chapter 2, there are 2 groups of individuals who use the word "healthy", and both groups use it to mean something different. Since very few people read true science or even understand true science, in this chapter the word "healthy" will refer to the low information group of people who seem to enjoy being fooled by politicians and who do not appear to want to be free of political influence.

To begin, there is absolutely no such thing as a healthy diet(medical term), or a healthy lifestyle, or a healthy supplement.

Sometime in the 1930s a scientist raised the question, "just how much must an organism consume in order to live"? Prior to this, how much Americans ate was influenced by politicians who supported the farmers of the US to sell their products. Someone came up with "3 square meals a day". I do not know who or when this occurred.

To continue, the scientist who questioned how much an organism required to live, raised a large collection of mice of similar genetics and placed them in multiple cages. I do not recall how many per cage, or how many cages. He then gave each cage a certain amount of food each day and recorded these amounts. He, like others, expected that the mice who received less food would live less time.

The cage that received the least amount of food, but just enough to not starve to death, lived the longest and they lived %30 more time than the cage just before them. Also autopsies on the mice revealed that this group of mice also suffered %50 less major illnesses than the other mice (diabetes, heart disease and cancers).

A group of scientists in Japan later repeated the same experiment and recorded the exact same results. This is what true science is. An experiment is designed to attempt to answer a question and the experiment can be repeated and the results recorded. It is not based on word of mouth or consensus (a vote). The numbers speak for themselves.

What the mice ate was not recorded as this was not a question the experiment designer was attempting to answer. So if an organism eats just enough to not die(noted in calories, or energy of the food), they will live the "healthiest" life (medical term). Nothing else is known about diet and health (medical) at this time.

The above experiment was performed on monkeys who had a short lifespan (about 15 years) and the same results were recorded.

The amount of activity or type of food was not recorded. So we do not know as of the publishing of this book, if what we eat, or how active we are has any effect on our health (medical). Weight also was not looked at as a factor. Only how many calories the organism consumed each day.

The mice were not given supplements. Just no food.

We Should All Practice by the Copernican Principal

How science can go wrong

Copernicus is most famously known for discovering and publishing his theory that the sun and not the earth, was the center of the known universe. However, his greatest contribution to the scientific world was his "Copernican Principal" which in simple terms, stated that no one and nothing is special in its existence. This allowed him to come up with his heliocentric theory and to see that the earth revolved around the sun.

The Copernican Principal can be used in all areas of science, including dentistry and medicine, and it should. When data is plotted such as time of death and amount of poison in the circulatory system, for example, one comes up with a bell shaped curve. A scientist can then assume that if your data falls within the bell shaped curve, it is a normal and not a special condition.

I will use an example of a simple bell shaped graph with age on the "y" or vertical axis, and weight on the "x" or horizontal axis. If a researcher were to plot the age and weight of a significant amount of people on this graph, he would discover that it makes a bell shaped curve. He can then assume that any points that fall within the bell shaped curve are considered to be normal. If outside the curve it can be considered to be abnormal or "special".

Illnesses that fall into this category include the flu. If a patient arrives at an office with a sore throat and a temperature, the physician only need imagine a bell shaped curve of what illnesses patients have been having the last month. If the flu is running rampant it would not make sense for the doctor to order blood tests to see if the patient has cancer or some rare illness from another continent.

Another of my favorites is the so called "strep throat". This phrase has come to mean a sore throat. The symptoms of strep throat last about 3 days. Very few if any patients will go to a doctor within the first 3 days of contracting a sore throat. But the physician will prescribe an antibiotic which throws the patient into a fungal infection. The patient then has a sore throat from candidiasis (a fungus). The physician (thinking the patient has a very bad bacterial infection)then gives a stronger antibiotic to the patient in an attempt to stop the sore throat. And all the physician has to do is remember what the most common cause of a sore throat is and use the Copernican principal to come up with a diagnosis, most likely of flu.

Fillings containing mercury can cause illness. I am convinced we can find a person in the world who will have an allergic reaction to every material the earth contains.

So a person can have an allergic reaction to a silver filling. But data demonstrates that mercury fillings do not cause illness.

In any population there will be a person who contracts thyroid cancer. If a nuclear power plant is in the area, the cancer will be blamed on that. Data shows this does not occur.

When a recommended cancer screening does not alter the number of persons contracting a disease such as cancer, instead of admitting the screening (preventive procedures) does not work, the physicians say the screening must be performed at an earlier age and more frequently.

These practitioners are not following the Copernican Principal, nor science. They are practicing consensus which will be discussed later.

Headaches, back aches and tooth aches

The symptoms in the title above are all best diagnosed using the Copernican Principal.

Stress is what I consider to cause most problems in human fitness. That is, stress causes most pains and some illness, data proves this. I simply have concluded this from 30 years of practice on patients and I have noted patterns in symptoms, treatment outcome, and patient attitudes. But, as I stated earlier, what is most important is that data (not my observations) demonstrate this.

There is data to show which diagnostic tools do not yield useful information in dealing with the above problems. Sometime in the 1990s, a study was conducted by military physicians and the purpose of the study was to determine if full body cat-scans or mri's could diagnose back problems or pains.

The study had a large sample (I remember around 10,000 subjects) and the way the study was conducted was that ½ of the physicians only used the full body cat-scans or mri's to perform the medical exam on new military recruites, ages 17-19. The other ½ of the physicians only performed a hands on exam of the same recruits.

The results of the experiment demonstrated that 90% of all healthy males aged 17-19 have distortions of the spinal column (vertebrae) and that these distortions are normal.

The physicians who only saw the cat-scans and mri's diagnosed 90% of the subjects to have major back problems needing surgery.

The physicians who only performed a physical exam on the subjects diagnosed only 5% (I can't recall the exact number) with back problems.

The above study without a doubt demonstrates that there is no diagnostic value of mri's or cat-scans or any back x-rays if a patient has back pains, unless the patient suffered trauma (a broken back) or has symptoms that might suggest a tumor in the spine.

And from this I move to people who suffer from headaches, tooth aches and neck aches. Stress causes a person to clench or grind their teeth(stress can be due to chemicals which then cause mental triggers, or simply psychological stress), mostly at night.

Many dental problems occur due to this, as clenching and grinding weaken teeth and this flexing of the tooth causes cavities to increase in size until the teeth are lost. It also drives patients to think they have "migraine" headaches which do not exist. Extreme headaches caused by clenching and grinding do exist. There is no mysterious condition termed a "migraine".

I do not know if dentists and physicians who pursue these symptoms as "migraines" are simply low information practitioners or if they don't want to admit their diagnosing and there fore "specialty" was ill conceived and therefore irrellevant.

My treatment is to simply reduce the stress. It can be achieved using chemicals(relaxation medications) or appliances in the mouth, or thru hypnosis. All are valid. But simply thinking that you must go to a physician to alleviate your pain can itself cause stress. Thinking that you must go to a doctor every 6 months in order to avoid pain causes stress. Thinking you are a patient your entire life can cause stress.

And why does this bother me? Because I must use my time to attempt to re-educate these patients who come to see me and want me to "desensitize" their teeth because another dentist did this in the past and told them this was the correct treatment, or to root canal a tooth because another dentist did this to a tooth and it worked for a while. Or they want to know how a tooth can still hurt if it was root canalled.

The answer to all the above is because the problem was not a bad tooth, but trauma to the teeth from clenching and grinding, caused by stress.

The Copernican Principal can diagnose the above symptoms if one is desired. If one were to graph all people with the above conditions one would find that stress causing bruxing or clenching would fall under the bell shaped curve. It is very unlikely that a person who experiences a headache has a tumor, for example. That is not to say no one gets tumors. But a good dentist should explain all to his patient and treat under the bell shaped curve.

Physicians think their job is to identify a condition which has a name and to treat this condition until it no longer has a name. They do not treat the patient.

Treatment should consist of accessing if a patient has intolerable pain or a condition which will shorten their expected life span AND the patient wants the pain or condition to stop.

Chapter Four

Of Blood Pressure Radiation, Cancer, Supplements, Cholesterol, Salt and Bacteria

This chapter is dedicated to the main evils of medicine, or so the medical professionals want us to believe. By evils I mean that these topics are what drives a medical practice and these topics keep most patients fearing for their lives instead of living their lives.

I first feel the need to tell you what my food pyramid is.

It consists of 3 items: Fat, Sugar and Salt. I need these 3 items in order to live and I love to eat foods with them in them. Until I see data that tells me they are not healthy(medical) I will continue to consume them as much as I desire because they make me happy and consuming them lowers my stress.

Now, back to the show:

Death by Association

Blood pressure as discussed earlier is not a disease. Blood pressure is what we need in order to be alive. The only reason to take a person's blood pressure is to be able to know if they are alive. No B.P. means not alive. Other than that, anything a medical professional tells you about blood pressure is fiction.

Our own government published data concerning BP and race in the US. According to their data, 33% of our population has high BP and should be treated. Really? 33% of our large population has an illness that will make them die younger than expected? Last time I checked, life expectancy has only increased each decade for the last thousand years except during war time. The data does not support their assumption.

The same with cholesterol. In an attempt to make things more simple, let me state that heart problems are NOT plumbing problems. The circulatory system is not like your irrigation system. It is not pumps connected to pipes. The circulatory system is a mass of tissue that acts to enable blood to flow in the body.

Double blind studies have been performed in the United Kingdom on patients who were experiencing heart pains, or angina. The physicians suggested heart bypass surgery, stating that arteries in the heart were 'clogged" much like your kitchen drain might be. So a wise researcher decided to find out if this was true.

The researcher decided to set up an experiment where all patients thought they were going to have surgery on their hearts in order to restore blood flow to the heart and remove the heart pain due to lack of oxygen. All patients received the same medications and even underwent general anesthesia and had incisions made and sutures placed so that none of the patients knew if they had received the surgery. The actual surgery was performed on only 50% of the patients.

This study was performed on a significant amount of patients (although I do not recall how many). The conclusions were that both groups had less heart pain. The bypass surgery did nothing for the patient. It was further concluded that heart pain was not due to lack of oxygen to the heart, but a chemical reaction to inflammatory chemicals in the blood stream. All the medicines given before and after the operations apparently lowered stress and inflammation.

I am not aware of any data that disproves the above. Now in the US I have heard on the radio, advertisements that bypass surgery will now be performed on "ALL" coronary arteries whether or not they are "clogged". For some reason it is very difficult for our society to understand and live by what the data shows. We all think "more" is better. So instead of practicing what indisputable data demonstrates, they instead increase their surgical recommendations.

I compare blood pressure to wrinkles in your skin. The older one is, the more wrinkles a person has. Same with blood pressure. The older you are, the higher reading a physician will get on his meter. Wrinkles are associated with death, but are not causal.

I mentioned earlier, that this book is meant for entertainment, although I know what I know and what I do not know.

I am not aware of a collection of data that has been peer reviewed and published that demonstrates that lowering blood pressure benefits a patient (i.e. prolongs their life), but there are papers with 10,000 or more data points (patients) that demonstrate clearly that lowering a patient's blood pressure does not benefit them at all. The physicians might as well tell you that if you remove all your wrinkles with plastic surgery that you will live longer, as people who have wrinkles are more likely to die.

A classic example of a scientist gone ignorant: An author (physician) performed a data search on blood pressure. He wanted to find if changing a person's blood pressure benefited a patient. His data showed clearly that it did not, that a patient's life expectancy was the same whether or not his blood pressure was lowered. The author then stated that since he gave his patients blood pressure medication for the last 30 years, he would continue to. Either he did not want to admit that he was mistreating patients, or he is really so ignorant that even when he authored a study, he was unwilling to go against pop-culture. Many scientists have been known to not go against their beliefs even though their intense training and education contradict those beliefs (Hitchens, "god is not GREAT").

Can you imagine, if highly trained scientists act this way, what is going on with our federal politicians? It is scary. This is what is driving the destruction of the US.

My favorite question to ask a physician is "is there any evidence or data that demonstrates that lowering a person's blood pressure benefits them"? I have never received anything close to a scholarly response. They all say "yes", as they look away from me. They seem to be irritated with me that I should question something that they do to all patients. They think I should just accept that everyone has their blood pressure taken and they don't ask if it benefits them, so why should I?

The NHANES fabricates health statistics for our government. Lately they reported that African Americans have a life expectancy of 74 years while people of European descent have a life expectancy of 79. They further reported that African Americans have higher resting blood pressure readings than European Americans. It is reports like this that add to incorrect conclusions about blood pressure.

There was no experimentation performed to see if the two statements above were causal, or simply associated with one another.

It most likely is a genetic trait that African Americans die sooner than European Americans, and that Africans have higher blood pressure. Simply statistics that have no other implication. Most medical professionals would draw the conclusion (incorrectly) that it is because of higher blood pressure that the Africans die sooner. This is incorrect science as no study of altering blood pressure in the groups was performed. These types of reports make medical professionals appear to be behaving as children, and this behavior is due to their having an agenda that is based on their beliefs.

Or I can say that mentally deficient medical professionals draw the wrong conclusions from data like the above.

Then why all the emphasis on B.P.? I wish I had an answer. I can only assume it is politics and/ or ignorance. No one wants to rock the boat. I will give you an example. I must use the parallel universe theory to demonstrate my point.

I will assume that there are two earths where all is the same except this: In universe "A" Joe is an 80 year old man with what institutions call high b.p. As a result his physician puts him on medication which lowers his blood pressure and gives the patient many side effects and makes him think about his condition for the rest of his short life. He can not go out of the house without thinking about taking his medication, or if he will die today.

In universe "b" Joe's physician does not take his b.p. and tells Joe, you are a little overweight, but if you are happy as you are, I am happy as well.

2 Years later, on the same day, same time, both Joes die of heart attacks. It seems that the b.p. medication and worrying did not change a thing. But in universe "b", Joe's relatives are angry that their uncle died and they want someone to pay for it. They retain a lawyer and sue the physician.

Remember in both universes all is the same except what the 2 physicians did. The physician in universe "B" was honest and based his treatment on facts and correct data. The patient enjoyed his life until his death. In universe "A", the physician based his treatment on what he saw on t.v. specials, what a drug salesman told him, and on how his colleagues treated similar patients.

In court, Joe B's attorney has a paid cardiac physician on the witness stand and the attorney asks him what the "standard of care" is in this caseold Same with global warming. The physician remarks that it is to give the patient blood pressure lowering medication. The physician's attorney then asks if there is any evidence that giving medication to lower blood pressure would have prolonged Joe's life. The cardiac physician simply says "of course".

The attorney, in his closing statement to the jury says" doesn't it make sense to give a patient blood pressure medication? Wouldn't you want your uncle to have this medication?"

The jury of course convicts the physician of malpractice and his insurance company must pay Joe's family a million dollars.

And now physicians in universe A and B prescribe blood pressure lowering medication to all their patients, not because there is any evidence that it benefits anyone, but because they do not want to be sued in a court. And so now we have attorneys deciding medical treatments based on how much money they can win in a law suite, and these conclusions are based on an uneducated and apathetic jury.

The worst part is that insurance companies and most government employers use blood pressure measurements to deny a person insurance or a job. The reasoning is that if you have high bp, you will require more medical services and medications to treat a condition that does not exist. Ironic, but true. It happened to me.

The miss-information exists in other illnesses as well. In the 1970's stomach cancer was all the rage. Organizations sponsored by the government placed advertisements on tv stating that drinking coke caused stomach cancer. I can only assume some politician did not like the Coca Cola company. There was never any data to support their efforts, and I guess the politicians gave up.

Lately the progressive administrations have been pushing restrictions on drinks that contain sugar. This too is aimed at the Coca Cola corp. If the liberal politicians cannot achieve their goals with one type of miss-information, they turn to another.

I compare the breast cancer scare to the global warming scare of present. As more information arose that performing breast cancer physical exams did not help at all in detecting breast cancer, the organizations who depend on keeping patients in fear in order to receive money from the government continued to change their tactics. Their goal was not to find the truth. Rather, it was to exist and receive government funds. The agencies changed their advertisements from "prevent breast cancer" to " breast cancer awareness". The agencies never told the public that going to a doctor to check for breast cancer did not benefit them.

Same with global warming. The only thermometer that existed before man existed was ice cores. These can determine the temperature of the earth at the time of their formation. But of local temperature only. Then the global fictionists (warming politicians) decided to scare people and decided they would say man was warming the planet. They did not tell anyone they were not using the same thermometer as existed before man's existence. They could not compare small temperature changes to the past. And the past ice cores demonstrated that the earth was much warmer before man, than it has been during man's existence. Also the cores demonstrated that carbon dioxide was not high when the temperatures were. So no the global alarmists are changing their tune and simply are saying carbon dioxide is a pollutant. They still then receive funding from the government. (I was wondering if I could sneak some global warming nonsense in here.)

To make things worse, only scientists whose goal it was to prove there was such a thing as global warming would receive funding from the government to perform their work. The same thing occurs in cancer studies.

The government wants us to view our bodies as Mr. Potato Heads, where each part is separate. They want us to think our bodies have plug in points where one can simply be removed and we are like new. Only then can they get support from the public to have funding for research and to justify their existence.

The cancer societies sponsored by our government, site as the main cause of cancer "radiation", and refer to data from the Nagasaki and Hiroshima nuclear explosions which ended World War II.

The data demonstrated that if a person where exposed to radiation outside the blast zone and radiation sickness zone, the survivors had less or similar cases of cancers as people who were not exposed to the radiation.

Even the sponsored data gatherers cannot alter the data from the Hiroshima and Nagasaki bomb blast survivors enough to support their propaganda that radiation causes cancer. The authors of these agenda reports suggest that there are errors in the collection of data, or that the higher rates of cancer will show up in the future.

These government supported "fake" scientists should be embarrassed to show their conclusions when the data clearly show the opposite. But our population is increasingly low information, and more of this will occur in the future.

Cancer is caused by genetics, virus and chemicals. That is what the data shows.

Salt was never found to decrease life expectancy. The story begins something like this:

In the early 1900's, a young doctor set out to see if there was any association with early death and salt intake. He visited an island with native people as he thought they would all be genetically similar and they most likely were. He then assumed that populations in the high lands had a smaller salt intake than those by the ocean shore, and he then took blood pressure readings. His results were that the population having higher bp readings lived closer to the coast. First of all, bp as I stated earlier is not a disease and does not cause earlier death. Second of all, living closer to the ocean does not mean higher salt intake. This is the only study I am aware of that attempts to connect salt intake and early death.

As the title of this section is "death by association", this is a great example of my statement. A wise physician stated (not me) that most conclusions so called scientists come up with, are associations which can be compared to this:

"When I wake up in the morning, the sun comes up".

These 2 events are associated but have no meaning or causal effect. That is what I call pop-culture. Low information people making scientific statements.

I recently read a research paper on facts. I think the title read "Facts in the US are dead". The study concluded that even with scientists, if they heard just 2 people who agreed with their points of view, they stored this view deep in their brains as facts, and that this opinion could not be changed by data.

The above is why I am attempting to teach scientists and others to follow facts and not consider consensus. To be "free thinkers" (Naryshkin, Evolution, Beliefs and Your Reality).

More is NOT Better

Many dentists and physicians prescribe antibiotics for the mythical heart murmur treatment, or other ailments because they have bought into the myth that more is better. That too is why the vitamin and supplement scams exist. If we need protein to live, them more must be better, right? Or what about water? Antibiotics?

Supplements—I do not know when it started, but someone came up with the idea that if you combine the ingredients of what humans are made of, that you somehow make a human. Problem is it doesn't work like that. But still, billions of people want to believe that it is so. These people take vitamins and supplements.

The only thing that studies on vitamins have demonstrated is that taking vitamins shortens a person's life. You will hear on the radio or tv that "studies show", but either there is no study, or it is not a real study. Recently I heard ads about a supplement that makes your cartilage grow in your joints. The supplement is made from chemicals similar to what the cartilage is made of.

Problem is that our body does not fabricate parts from parts. If that was so, our mother would have to eat a brain in order for us to have a brain, a heart for us to have a heart, etc.

There is no science to back up supplements or vitamins. A person would have to be severely restricted in their diet in order to need supplemental vitamins in order to grow or function correctly. I am aware of only 2 times in history when this is known to have occurred and both were during war time.

Radiation—This phenomenon was relatively unknown until WWII when the United States fabricated and used 2 nuclear bombs on Japan to end WWII. I imagine this is where the horror stories of radiation and cancer were formed.

Nuclear radiation at high energy, such as is released in a nucler explosion, obliterates everything at close range. At intermediate distances people died of radiation poisoning, which is not cancer, but the death of rapidly reproducing cells in the body which leads to the patients bleeding to death. Outside of this zone people received only radiation burns.

Since the time of the nuclear bombs, various agencies have attempted to perform studies on survivors. Independent studies wanted to see what long term effects the radiation in the outer region of the bombs had on people. Government agencies wanted to scare the populace into thinking that radiation in the outer region caused cancer.

If one were to find a government sight on cancer and the causes of cancer (remember it is all propaganda), you would find that they list radiation as the primary cause of cancer. They even list their evidence to be the Hiroshima and Nagasaki bombs.

And no one wants to rock the boat as the new "fact" is to go along with the crowd (pop culture).

The results, based on data, show that radiation does not cause cancer, and in fact has a protective effect on people. Government sponsored studies (which had agendas) still showed no higher cancer rates, but the publishers put disclaimers in the reports stating that they thought not enough time had passed to show an increase in the amount of cancer. Why the US government has an agenda to prove radiation causes cancer, I do not know, but I am sure it is connected to politics.

Dental x-rays have never caused cancer in a patient. Even dentists from the earliest x-ray machines who held the film in their hands and received massive doses of x-radiation, did not conceive cancer. Some did get ugly growths on their fingers, but no cancer.

Studies of women who received high doses of x-radiation to the chest in order to fight tuberculosis showed lower rates of breast cancer than the general public.

To add to this, I was pleasantly surprised when I found that even state health departments do not require the use of dental lead aprons when taking x-rays on patients as there was no evidence of any danger to the patient. The use of a dental lead apron for x-rays was purely cultural, and adds to the incorrect assumption that x-rays are dangerous.

Chapter Five

Is There Such a Thing as Preventive Medicine?

No.

Vaccines can prolong life.

Ridding a body of parasites can prolong life.

Visiting the doctor every 6 months does NOT prolong life. 60 years ago physicians were taught that longevity was directly tied to one's income. No one questioned this for years. Then an actual study was performed about 1980 and surprise! No connection between longevity and income. No connection between access to physicians and longevity.

This is one of the greatest lies to the general public ever made. And I think this arose from the 1940's when unions could not increase a union members pay, so to attract new employees the unions offered medical insurance and they competed for propaganda. One thing that made prospective members desire their insurance was that it paid for exams every 6 months(medical and dental). This time frame was not based on science but on propaganda. And then the general public adopted this as a necessary part of their lives.

As I stated earlier, studies demonstrated that longevity was not connected in any way to access to medical care (including exams).

Heart attacks are not due to a plumbing problem. I have concluded after observing many reports on data that heart attacks are due to inflammatory products in the circulatory system that are fabricated by our bodies when under chemical stress that can be brought on by psychological stress which is transferred to chemical stress. Inflammation can be due to only chemical stress itself. How this is done I do not know. I only know the big picture.

A recent study concluded that more people suffer strokes and heart attacks if that person lives closer to areas which experience high noise which it is assumed causes more stress. Even though the above study backs up my statements of inflammation causing heart attacks,

I consider the data to be anecdotal. I think more of a controlled study has to be performed before it can be said for sure that this is what occurs.

Our government has now begun funding to societies in order to demonstrate that sugar causes inflammation. This is not science as it has an agenda. If they really cared about people they would be funding studies on "what" causes inflammation.

In addition to the above, fitness does not add to longevity. Circumstantial evidence I have observed (not scientific data) demonstrates that greater physical activity does not prolong a person's life. If there were data to demonstrate that people who exercised lived longer, it would have to be shown that the exercise caused this. It could be that a person simply felt better if they were to live longer and so exercised. But there is no evidence of this.

There is also data that demonstrates that long distance runners or joggers over the age of 45, have higher rates of heart failure than non-runners.

And what would the value be of living longer? The proponents of living longer show no evidence that it prolongs your life in the 20s or 30s. As far as I can see, it prolongs your life in the 80s or 90s. Is that a good thing?

I will play devil's advocate and for discussion sake and assume if one were to take vitamins, and exercise and eat only grass that you will add 2 years to your life. Will it have been worth it to worry every day of your life if you took the correct vitamins that day? Would it be worth it for you to have thought about your next physicians visit and if he would find cancer on you? Would it be worth it for you to have spent the time and money on those visits and supplements and treatments rather than on a really relaxing vacation? Only to live 2 more years in a diaper in a nursing home?

I argue that it is not.

What a medical examination is for—a medical examination is to allow the physician to document the decay of a human being, and for the doctor to gather evidence on you in case in the future you decide to sue him for neglect.

A parent takes his child to see a doctor for a visit. Pediatricians examine children for the same reasons.

First of all, it is called a "wellness" exam, as that is the pop-culture phrase that apparently parents accept. Many parents do question why they are persuaded to take a child who is not sick, to the doctor. I imagine it is difficult to say no to a wellness exam for your child.

A pediatric exam mainly consists of measuring and weighing the child and taking his temperature. And just what does this accomplish? Nothing. Again, it is documenting evidence in case you were to sue the physician in the future. It has nothing to do with your child. You can not follow a curve on a graph to decide how much to feed your child, nor should you. It is just a collection of data that the doctor can present in court if you sue him. He can say, "but your honor, our measurements demonstrate that the child was growing at a normal rate."

To conclude; a pediatric exam (children's exam) is designed for you to pay a doctor to collect data to be used against you in case of a legal suite. It is insane. And we do it

And What of Longevity?

3 anecdotal stories

1. A study of which country contained the most centenarians. Results—Cuba. What all the centenarians had in common—they all smoked at least one cigar a day and drank at least one cup of coffee a day.
2. Longevity of WWII concentration camp survivors—a large amount (how many I do not know) lived to be over 90 years old. In common? They all underwent a prolonged time of near starvation.
3. Oldest living human as of 2013. A man in Chile was 123 years old. What did he do? He did not visit the doctor, he ate potatoes every day, and chewed coco leaves every day.

So are any of these people's life habits or diets ever mentioned on tv or the internet? I think not. Although all of the above are anecdotal (they were not studies), they do occur. My conclusion is that starvation is the only thing that prolongs life, but taking part in rituals involving chemicals which relax you makes your life worth living. If you are not relaxed, and able to enjoy your life, then why live at all?

Anything else that the government tells us about health is a lie. It is said only for political reasons. They know now that if they tell our population that something is more "healthy", most people will believe that it is true and that it means medical health.

We are "over" nourished. It is healthy(medical term) to be "under" nourished. One bowl of cereal (cherios) has enough vitamins and minerals for us to survive on for a week.

What about gyms?—as far as the data shows, anything that involves activity lessens a person's life expectancy. There is no data to say otherwise. Anecdotal evidence shows that professional and Olympic athletes die younger than non-athletes. A small study recorded data that showed that people who run past the age of about 45 have a higher rate of heart attack than non-runners. The "why" is not known yet, but the "is it good for longevity" is known, and it is a solid "no".

Not allowing a person to take an alchoholic drink a day, or to injest a chemical such as tobacco or other, causes stress which causes disease which can shorten a persons life or at the least, make it not be enjoyable.

And no magical food or supplement has been found to be needed in order to live. I do think that if a person is to perform the starvation diet in order to prolong his life, he must eat a hole food on occasion. Whole foods (such as eggs) contain everything a person needs to grow normally. I do not recall all whole foods, but something as simple as eating a cockroach every week would most likely supply your body with all that was needed.

What you need or require to live has not been calculated. Whole foods have all of what is needed to grow an entire human being. I do not know where the data lies concerning whole foods. Yet I am convinced it is so.

Salt is one of those nonsense things. There is no evidence at all that eating salt makes you die younger. No studies have been conducted to determine this. And all people require salt in order to live. But the media and hence, doctors, have adopted a war on salt. With no medical evidence that it increases or decreases your health(medical). None.

I worked in a autopsy room when I was 18 years old and observed and participated in about 100 autopsies. Although not research or enough data points to satisfy data, I observed one patient to be 40 years old who died of a heart attach as told by observers. He was in fantastic physical shape and no plaques were found in his heart blood vessels.

Another patient was 86 and also died of a heart attack. His coronary arteries were filled with a white buttery substance. I think that if he went to a physician every 6 months his doctor would have ordered him to take cholesterol lowering meds and to exercise. And for what? Remember, he was 86! How long are we supposed to live?

And the 40 year old would have been told he was very healthy.

My point is that preventive medicine does not exist and believing that there is such a thing only causes stress in a person which lessens his enjoyment of life.

12 year wonders

These are items or topics that seem to appear every 12 years. The best excuse I have heard for this recurrence of stories, is that the generations these topics hit are the youngest and that the media waits about 12 years to put stories out on these again so it can attract a new audience who was too young to remember the story when it last came around.

My favorite recurring story is the one about salmonella bacteria in raw eggs. My grandfather, father and I all ate raw eggs. My grandfather was a chicken farmer as was I. When I was in my athletic years the market for powdered proteins did not yet exist, so I ate raw eggs. I never did get any salmonella infections and I never met anyone who did. This is just anecdotal, not science as I did not study the subject and collect data.

But the story for some reason died out about a month later not to be seen again until my college days, then about every 12 years thereafter. If it is a real problem, then why does the story always go away? This ongoing drama is a fabrication of politics and the media.

Exposure to the sun causes skin cancer. Or so they say. Physicians and politicians have been attempting to pull this one on us for years. There never was any data to suggest exposure to the sun caused skin cancer or melanoma. The only data I am aware of shows that since the use of protective skin creams have been in wide use, the incidents of skin cancer have increased. This tells me it is chemicals and not the sun causing the cancer.

The more serious cancer physicians attempt to connect to the sun is melanoma. Strange that it often originates on the buttocks or in the mouth.

Breast cancer advertisements were all over tv in the 1970s-1980s. Women were told to have their breast manually examined by physicians, and to have breast x-rays (mammograms) taken. They were told that the more breast exams they had, the more likely they were to not die of breast cancer. Then along came a report from the UK with a large amount of data points (patients). The suggestion of the authors was that if a woman has not had a female family member who was diagnosed with breast cancer, the woman should never have a mammogram, as she would only receive false readings from the exams.

As a result, in the US we do not see the advertisements any more. The US government sponsored societies will not admit they were wrong. Instead they have reworded their efforts to "breast cancer awareness". I imagine this is so they can continue to scare women into thinking they are going to die of breast cancer.

I liken the US governments attempt to scare us about breast cancer to it's attempt to scare us about skin cancer. For many decades we were all told to not go outside unless we had suntan lotion on. After decades these studies have shown that the more we used suntan lotion, the more skin cancer we got. So we don't see many government commercials about using suntan lotion anymore. But no apologies. Did the lotion cause the cancer? We will never be told.

One more example of how politics effects cancer doctrine: In the 1970s, a political group which protects animals at the expense of humans concluded, not from science, but from anecdotal stories, that frogs were being found with abnormalities in their lymbs. This group then concluded that these malformations were the result of genetic mutations from higher than normal levels of the sun's rays which was due to a hole in the ozone layer of our atmosphere, and that this hole was caused by humans using Freon in their airconditioners.

From the above, they then concluded that humans would soon be getting genetic mutations from the sun and that we must wear protective sun screens in order that we not get basal cell carcinoma or the deadly "melanoma".

In the same manner that associations took off with the heart murmur debacle, these groups provided much ammunition for the progressives to convince people that they were evil and were causing harm to animals and that we would all get cancer if we did not follow their strict instructions.

So for a few decades, we were flooded with instructions on how to use sun protection. It was just like the radiation scare from WWII.

Sometime in the 1990's, some scientists(who actually were scientists), discovered that the defects in the frogs were not from radiation at all. That a fungus was causing this.

On top of this, melanoma was never connected to sun exposure, as melanoma can form where the sun don't shine, even in the mouth. But with our pop-culture communication and government propaganda, these things just take off and as I stated earlier, even physicians will back up their beliefs rather than search for sound data.

One of my greatest frustrations is that even those who graduate with science degrees do not understand what science is. My favorite example is the myth that stretching before exercising prevents injuries. In the 1970s an article was published in the Sports Medicine Journal (at least that is what I think the journal was called). In the research the authors were very diligent in stating their limits of the research and of how the study was conducted. Their conclusion was that the data showed that stretching in deed did not have any effect on injury to the athlete.

But time marches on, and in 2011 I read an article of a very similar if not similar title and it was published in a sports journal, although I can not recall the name of the journal. I do, however, recall that the article from the 1970s was not sighted in the recent article. So these 2011 researchers were in fact redoing research that was very well examined in the 1970s. The authors did not perform a standard literature review of past studies. Had they performed this they would have discovered that the research had already been performed.

This is an example of how little scientists pay attention to research.

The same conclusions were attained in the newer study as in the original. But what a waste of time and research. It is but another example of how ignorant even researching scientists are.

I suspect that activity lessens longevity because it causes a person to consume more, and all we know so far is that consuming less makes us live longer. But it must be starvation, not just a few less calories.

And what about supplements? The only data where research was conducted using supplements or vitamins as the variable, recorded earlier deaths if daily vitamins were taken versus placebos. There is no data from peer reviewed studies which demonstrate a longer life with the use of vitamins or supplements.

You will often read or hear that supplement "a" is healthy and is now 100% stronger than before! Problem is that, if there is a published paper to back this up, it is a paper in which the author did not refer to any significant data, and the reader gets all excited about "is it really 100% stronger?," rather than looking into "is there really any data that demonstrates that substance "a" makes us live longer with less major illness?

The authors who think they are scientists and think that they are publishing a scientific paper use references which use other papers of what people say, not of what does the data show?

In the 1970s, the news media was giving people daily lists of what can give your car more gas mileage. It came to an end when an intelligent journalist finally decided to add up all the recommended actions. He found that if you followed all the advice on t.v., your car would actually be creating gasoline. For example, a tune up might give you 20% more mileage, new tires 30%, etc. The total savings combine for over 100%.

The same thing can be said of the lists that currently are given to people to prolong their life. I am surprised to see that no one has yet added them up to see that the math proves these fads do not work. And the claims are made with no data. The claims are said to come from "4 out of 5 doctors recommend", etc. It is ignorance run amuck. We value what someone thinks more than what the research or data shows.

My thoughts on pediatrics

Life is natural. A plants grows from a seed. Birds hatch from eggs. Why is the birth of a human looked at as if major surgery is being performed on a person to remove a tumor?

I have no problem with having an ob/gyn at the birth of my child. He is there for an emergency. If something goes wrong it must be fixed immediately or permanent damage can occur to your child. It is the rest that I have a problem with.

Decades ago a parent was encouraged to change their child's diaper in the hospital. If the child cried, it was hungry and the parent gave the child a bottle of formula.

Flash forward to the current day. A parent cannot change a child's diaper for fear that if something goes wrong, the parent might sue the hospital. If a child cries, the parent may not give a bottle of formula until the nurse sticks the child and draws some blood to be tested for blood sugar level. Only then can a bottle of formula be given and only by the nurse. A parent does not need a blood test to see if a child is hungry. It all goes back to the staff preparing for a law suite. They can write a number down to prove a child has enough nutrition. The child is treated as a "specimen" that the parents must not touch and it is all done for the sake of a future law suite.

Parents blindly take their children to the pediatricians office and the help measures, weighs and takes the temperature of the child. This is all done (once again), in case of a law suite. They can argue that on that day, at that time the child did not have an abnormal temperature or weight. There is no other reason as only a very unobservant parent would not notice something was wrong with their child.

And now the pediatric staff attempt to make children into vegetarians. I ate what I wanted when I was a child (and still do) and I turned out fine. There is no evidence that being a vegetarian is good for a child or adult. It is all political propaganda. I resist anything our federal government suggests, and so should you.

On vaccines, I have not seen any data that would suggest vaccines harm a child. But I argue that a child should not be vaccinated for hepatitis B until he is older. I was shocked to find that hospitals want parents to just accept that their child be injected with hepatitis B vaccine the day he is born. A child has little if no risk of obtaining hepatitis B infection. Again, this a political propaganda thing.

I discuss in the next chapter on dentistry what is important about fluoride, and the pediatricians do not prescribe this, and fluoride would prevent dental decay in the adult teeth at this stage.

Chapter Six

Dental

Fluoride! Fluoride! Fluoride!

If you don't know why you are doing

something, don't do it!

Dental Myths

Wisdom teeth should be extracted

Cleaning your teeth gets rid of bad breath

Wisdom teeth make your teeth crooked

Brushing too hard makes grooves in your teeth

Pains in teeth means you have a cavity or need a root canal

Gum disease causes heart disease

Big needles hurt more than small needles

Myths (continued)

Warm anesthetic (numbing solution) hurts less than room

temperature liquid

Sealants prevent tooth decay (cavities).

If you have a heart murmur you must take a large dose of antibiotics before having any dental work performed on you.

A pocket in the gums must be treated.

Being that I am a dentist, this section will have some very specific information that might only interest dentists.

Here are some categories as to why a patient chooses to see the dentist. They are 1. For prevention. 2. For decay. 3. For gum disease. 4. For traumatic damage to teeth(broken teeth).5. Cosmetics

I will be sure to address these in this chapter.

Dentistry is concerned with less important procedures than medicine, but since I am a dentist I will critique my profession. For those dentists who might be offended by my criticism, I want to say that I am not perfect, and my criticism is not about errors that anyone can make, or criticism of artistic technique. My critique is about members of our profession who do not follow science. There is no excuse to not prevent injury to your patient before their butt hits the chair.

General safety—One of the most performed procedures in dentistry is the injection. When needles are designed, a designer does not simply draw a pointed instrument and say "that's it"!. He must consider many things. These include, what is the purpose of the needle?, what is needed in order to perform the procedure?, is it safe?.

First, the needle must be able to deliver the intended chemical to the intended sight. So the needle must have a minimum inner diameter as too small a diameter will not allow the fluid to flow. The needle must be of adequate length to reach desired anatomical areas.

The needle must cause no harm. Early studies revealed that too thin a needle can flex when inserted into tissues and that this can sever nerves and blood vessels. So the needle must be able to resist flexing. The needle must not break under the tissue as it is very difficult to retrieve when under soft tissue. The needle must be of adequate inner diameter to allow aspiration(suction of blood into the syringe so the operator can view if he is in a vessel) of blood so the dentist can know if he is in a blood vessel.

Pain is not a consideration as studies have shown that a person cannot distinguish when a thin or thick needle is used for an injection. Patients simply do not like needles in their mouths.

As a result of the above considerations, the 25 gauge long needle was found to be the minimum thickness and length of needle dentists should use in order to minimize risk of injury to a patient. And the 23 gauge is recommended on children(McDonald, Ralph E. 1983). This is not only in published studies, but it is taught in good dental schools across the country.

What occurs—every dentist with the exception of one, that I have come into contact with uses either a 30 or a 27 gauge needle. When I ask them why, they freeze and either say nothing or say "I don't want to hurt my patient". So they do not know why they are using an instrument they are licensed to use. There is no thinking or consideration in deciding their choice.

An injection of an anesthetic into a blood vessel in the head and neck area can travel back towards the brain and cause seizures. I have been a witness to this on 2 occasions, when the dentists used 27 instead of 25 gauge needles.

Too short and thin a needle can cause a break in the needle under the soft tissue. I am aware of 2 dentists who did this and both denied their mistake and blamed it on the company who manufactured the needles.

As an air force pilot, I was trained to always follow a strict protocol and to be responsible for my actions. I was not trained to perform a maneuver in an aircraft because a manufacturer or friend told me to. It was not consensus that ruled, but instruction based on data from test pilots. The same can be said of dentistry and it's techniques, but dentists decided they know better because their dental supply representative told them it was ok.

And almost every 6 months I hear from a patient that they are too sensitive to epinephrine for it to be used on them. This simply means the dentist injected the anesthetic solution into a blood vessel due to him not aspirating with a 25 gauge or larger needle. Injection of epinephrine into a blood vessel will cause a patient to shake.

The most severe result I have witnessed as the result of a dentist using too thin a needle is the severing of the nerve that feeds the lower jaw. So ill informed are dentists that there was an episode where a dentist (perhaps a few) experienced paresthesia (permanent nerve damage) to the lower jaw of their patients while injecting them. The dentists blamed this on the anesthetic rather than their injection techniques and even published a paper stating that the brand of anesthetic they used mysteriously damages only the nerve to the lower jaw and so should not be used for those injections.

It was found from independent review and observations of the above patients that the dentists were using small diameter needles (not 25 gauge) and that they were using poor injection technique and that they had mechanically severed the patient's nerves from trauma of the needle. The dentists apparently were oblivious to the fact that they were not using correct equipment or technique and that it "must" be the anesthetic solution.

Either the dentists attended very poorly run dental schools or they were following the low information consensus technique our society proposes. (they listened to their low information friends rather than what the research shows).

I have also been aware of 2 cases personally where a dentist broke a thin needle off under the soft tissue of a patient and then had to have the patient almost dissected alive in order to remove the needle. These were completely avoidable situations.

While on the subject of injections, I will talk about the temperature of the anesthetic. A study just as meticulously carried out as the thickness of the needle test(patients were injected with both incorrect thin needles and the correct 25 gauge without their knowledge) demonstrated that a patient does not have less discomfort during an injection if the liquid is heated to body temperature nor if the needle is large or small gauge.

Even though there is no evidence that the temperature of the anesthetic changes the sensation of an injection, I have seen low information dentists placing their anesthetic cartridges in a heating device or placing them against their skin under their glove in the "belief" that they are being more caring towards their patient, when in fact they are only spreading misinformation to the public.

Most wisdom teeth do not have to be removed and should not be removed. Again, we are taught this in dental school but when the low information dentists get out into a practice they panic and do what the other dentists around them are doing.

A wisdom tooth only must be removed 1. If it is causing inflammation or pain, 2. If it's being there is causing decay on the adjacent tooth,3. If the orthodontists wants to pull the adjacent tooth back in the jaw.

A wisdom tooth is like an appendix or gall bladder. We do not remove these just because on some people they can cause a problem. And removing a wisdom tooth can often result in permanent damage to the nerve that runs through the lower jaw, and painful healing.

Still, I hear many dentists tell patients they need their wisdom teeth removed. They do not cause your teeth to be crowded and crooked. All data demonstrates this.

Blood thinners. For some reason dentists think they must take a patient off blood thinners before performing dental procedures. While I question the value of putting a patient on blood thinners for any reason, the data shows that if a patient is removed from a blood thinner for a dental procedure, there is a great risk of stroke or heart attack, more so than if they were never on a blood thinner. This risk is greatest on the 3rd day of being removed from the blood thinner which is when the dentist usually starts his dental procedure.

I have had dentists rationalize that they think the patient will bleed longer after an extraction or gum procedure if on blood thinners. And I respond with the fact that not one patient has ever bled to death from being on a blood thinner during a dental procedure or after, but plenty have had heart attacks or strokes as a result of coming off the thinners. I have this knowledge from research articles published in the

Academy of General Dentistry. And I was taught this by knowledgeable oral surgeons while attending dental school.

Gum Disease: This is a confusing topic for patients, and dentists. Because scaling and root planning until no pocket over 3 millimeters exists, makes money, all dentists and hygienists do their best to get a measurement over this during their exam and they then hold their chest out proudly as they just brought in some big money to the practice.

Problem is, most pockets do not have to be treated. Data does not show that gum disease causes heart disease. In fact, in the data from the study on heart murmurs (100,000 data points), it can be concluded that it does not. Stress causes systemic inflammation which causes gum disease and heart disease. But telling a patient this does not make money for the office. (I am not against making money. I am just against making money at the expense of a patient's body).

Also, when a patient is given a systemic anti-inflammatory, both systemic inflammation and gum disease go away, with or without dental treatment.

Gum pockets are good to treat when performing cosmetic dentistry as the dentist does not want his new veneer to look ugly after it is placed. This can happen if the patient has pockets and the tooth associated with that pocket is prepared for a crown or veneer. If the gum is agitated, which often occurs from the drill or impression and temporary coverage fabrication, the gum can shrink towards the bone and expose the root. If the gum is treated prior to this, the shrinking will take place prior to the fabrication so the result covers this ugly root.

Sealants. A sealant is a thin layer of filling material to be placed in the grooves of teeth for the purpose of preventing tooth decay (cavities). Sounds good in theory. Only problem is, the data does not back this up.

There are many reasons why this does not work. First of all, if a tooth did not receive enough fluoride while developing, it will get decay if sealed or not as the sealant does not cover the entire tooth.

If the sealant were to work as theorized, it would not work, as dentists do not use correct technique in placing them. The grooves in the teeth must be drilled to remove any debris, and the surface must be etched with a chemical for at least 2 minutes on baby teeth, something I have never observed in an office. The sealant then fails.

To make things worse, most offices have an assistant perform sealant placement, not the dentist. The tooth is not kept dry, which is necessary for any composite material (which sealants are, to adhere to the tooth. But sealants are treated as a tooth cleaning. Why should anyone object? And since most insurances will pay the dentist for this, it is a sure way to make more money.

Once again, it is a procedure to make money, not make life better for the patient.

Much of the above errors are forced by the way dental practices are now run.

Instead of a dentist guiding the ship, most offices have an office manager who lives on commissions of what the patient pays to the practice.

The dentist walks into an office and the office manager tells him that this or that is what is expected of him if he is to keep his job there. Many dentists who succeed in these types of practices will brag to colleagues of how much commission they received, not of how well their patients are treated.

You see, the dentists act on what they think their colleague will say, rather than on what they know, or what the data shows.

Heart Murmurs and Bacteria

Before I begin, I want to state that the human body cannot be sterilized. I have read from one biologist, that the human organism contains more "non-human" bacterial cells than human cells. I do not have any data nor the way in which the biologist collected his data. But I sense that it is true if not close to factual.

The bacteria of the body live in harmony with other bacteria and their host (the body they live in). Problems only occur when the collection of bacteria is no longer in balance (when more of one bacteria now occupies an area where 2 or 3 equally shared the space).

It is very uncommon for a person to receive bacteria from an outside source that is not normally in the human body. But as soon as someone coughs they think they have a bacterial infection which requires antibiotics to cure. And physicians and dentists buy into this story as it is easier to go along with the crowd and give the audience what they want, or perhaps some physicians and dentists just really don't understand microbiology. As I stated earlier, using the Copernican principal here would remove a lot of the useless prescription writing, but might lessen an office's income.

Almost every odd thing a person experiences (a sore on the finger, a swollen gum, a sore throat) is from a virus or the person's own bacteria.

Heart murmurs. One of my favorite subjects because I was taught the truth as a student and then have had to fight it out with every dentist I have since met due to them all adopting what other misinformed dentists have told them, rather than follow or know what the research shows.

There was never any connection made between bacterial growths forming on damaged heart valves, from dental work. There was never any connection made between taking a strong antibiotic before dental work and having a lesser chance of getting bacterial growths on a damaged heart valve. However, our dental associations and dentists, for some reason "believed" that there was.

And remember that associations, or political parties care about their existence, not the people they claim to be helping.

Recently (the last 10 years or so) new reports have come to light about heart disease. The report claimed that there was an association between heart disease and gum disease. And I discussed previously about death by association. Association usually is not causal.

The heart and dental associations jumped right on this report and hijacked it to say that gum disease causes heart disease.

It took the American Heart Association about 70 years to admit their claims about heart murmurs were based on anecdotal stories and non-scienctific data. They had to find a reason to exist and they have once again found a reason for people to donate money to their cause.

I argue that inflammation in the body causes heart disease and gum disease. They both occur due to a systemic inflammatory reaction. I do not have data to back this up directly, but I have not come across any data to connect gum disease to heart disease. There are only reports that contain "he said" in them. The research from the Brazil/UK study on heart murmurs already concluded that bacteria from the mouth has not been associated with heart disease.

Based on the past history of what Americans will believe, it will take at least 70 more years for the fraudulent story asserting that gum disease causes heart disease to be put to rest.

Dental Franchises

(or Deceit and Intimidation Centers)

And now we come to the dental franchises. I consider these to be the major downfall of dentistry. They are discount stores in which the top of the pyramid is not the dentist, but the office manager who acts as top sales person.

The dentist is valued below janitor as the patients are brainwashed into thinking that you can order what you want from a menu and if they do not get it, the dentist is to blame.

No longer is the dentist the diagnostician and designer of treatment plans. Rather, what occurs in these establishments is this.

1. The patient arrives at the office and his insurance is checked to see what he can get without paying. The office is sure he will not reject this.
2. He then walks into a room with an assistant who takes a full set of x-rays. I stated earlier that x-rays do not cause cancer, but they do cost money. They

are taken to build a defense against a future law suite, and to find things to sell to the patient. This is not correct protocol in most states in the laws that govern a dentists' license. Only the dentist can order x-rays. But these establishments put the patients into a conveyor belt designed to bring in the most money. It is not designed to give the patient the best treatment.

3. To make things worse, the patient next gets pushed to the hygienist who once again cannot diagnose, treatment plan nor prescribe treatment for a patient. So how did the patient get first to the assistant for x-rays, and second, to the hygientist for a prophy or other gum treatment? I guess it works the same way our politicians do things. The politicians can go against the constitution as long as no one calls them on it. The same in dentistry. Patients don't know a dentist must see them and order treatments first.

4. Even if the dentist tells a patient a treatment will not work, the patient will not believe him. The patient looked at his menu before coming to the

office and the assistant and or hygienist agreed with him and added more on to his treatment because they get a commission. At the end, the manager sells all the stuff the assistant and hygientist sold him, even though legally they cannot, and for good reason!

5. When the patient shows up for further treatment he usually is treated by another dentist who is in on it all and does what the patient paid for whether or not it can work or last more than a day.

6. The dentist must use the laboratory chosen by the franchise owner. These laboratories are usually based in China and use materials that most likely are not real (i.e. metals that do not contain gold, or platinum) and who knows what chemicals as reactants or solvents. And a lot of what makes a dental practice successful is the dentist and laboratory's ability to work together. I change my laboratory every time I find one that is able to do a better job. I do not blame the laboratory if a bad result is achieved on a crown or denture. It is just that the laboratory and I did not work well

together. In a franchise that choice of the dentist to find a laboratory he works well with is taken away.

7. Then the dentist and staff must lie to the patient and tell them there is a laboratory fee added to their crown or denture due to the expense when their laboratory is most likely the least expensive in the country.

8. The dental office is a convenience store where tooth brushes and mouthwash are pushed on the customer.

The way it should be done:

1. A patient shows up for his appointment and tells the front desk he is there. He fills out a questioner about his medical problems.

2. He is seated in a dental chair and the dentist arrives and asks the patient what he wants. Does he have a specific problem? Does he want a full check up so the dentist can see if he finds anything wrong?

3. The dentist tells (prescribes) to the assistant what if any x-rays he wants.

4. The dentist performs his exam using the x-rays as added information.

5. The dentist diagnoses problems and devises treatment plans which can repair what the patient needs and wants. The last treatment option always is "do nothing".

6. The patient can then decide if he desires to follow the dentists' treatment plan (one of them) and appointments are made. One of these appointments usually is a hygiene appointment the dentist prescribes.

3 Beneficial Things Your Dentist Should Do Before Your Butt Hits The Chair.

I include these as these are items that are very important in protecting you against injury in the dental office.

1. Decide to only use 25 gauge long needles on all patients.
2. Do not prescribe a patient any type of antibiotic pre-medication for heart murmurs.
3. Do not tell a patient to stop taking blood thinners for any dental procedure if he is taking them.

Classic dentistry is dead

By "classic dentistry" I speak of the dentistry I was taught by my wise and experienced instructors. By classic dentistry I mean dentistry which involves the dentist being the aircraft commander of the office and patient, as it should be.

Classic dentistry does not fit into pop culture. It is not "fluff". It involves a caring and experienced dentist who takes pride in his diagnosis and treatment planning. He wants his patients to be pain free and their teeth to be functional for as long as possible. The only institutions in which I can confidently say this occurs is the military. Of course there are many veterans who will complain of military dental treatment, but these complainers are patients who are believers in pop culture, who believe x-rays and silver fillings are bad for you. The dentists in the military are straight shooters and want to get the soldiers they treat in working condition for as long as possible. That is their goal. It is not how much money they can get from a patient by selling them fluff as a salesman might sell them.

Fluoride—This is definitely the most important item a dentist can give a young patient or pregnant mother.

30 years ago the importance of fluoride was drilled into us in dental school and I observed first hand the protective effects of systemic fluoride on tooth decay. I worked in clinics in which a majority of the patients were children. The best thing a parent can do for their child is to not subject them to dental treatment of any kind. The only way to achieve this is for the mother to take oral fluoride while pregnant so that the fluoride is part of every baby tooth. The child will never get tooth decay in it's baby teeth.

The next step is to give the child systemic oral fluoride 2-3 days per week until age eight so that his adult teeth will not have any decay.

It is during this age(birth to 8 years old) that the enamel of the adult teeth are forming and the fluoride will be incorporated into the adult tooth structure.

Since I am writing this book as entertainment, I will leave it up to you to find the suggested dose of fluoride to give your child. Even if your water is fluoridated, take the fluoride as the children sometimes do not drink water.

All an overdose will do is perhaps slightly darken their teeth, but they will not decay. I have only seen badly colored teeth (called fluorosis) in cases where the child was raised on well water that had too much natural fluoride in it.

A child can overdose on fluoride if he were to drink an entire bottle of fluoride at a sitting. You must then call poison control. This, does not make fluoride a dangerous item to avoid.

The Mechanics of Dentistry

Another area of dentistry in which dentists do not follow the data is in the mechanics of dentistry. This involves judgment in observing if there is enough tooth structure to support what the dentist is planning. Think of this subject as one of engineering.

For a tooth to be restored, it must have enough sound tooth structure which means hard, non-decayed structure. Filling materials cannot take all the forces of chewing or grinding. These limitations are taught to us in dental school and are based on dental researchers using engineering devices to test the strength of different materials when restoring teeth. Dentists seem to throw this information away as soon as a salesman arrives at their office and gives them a free sample of some material.

The most errors in judgment I have seen have to do with root canals. If the tooth does not have enough tooth structure to be restored with a crown the tooth should not be root canalled as it will simply crumble in short time. I do not want to go into details here as it will not help the average patient and dentists can review their texts to find what these limits are. As I have stated in this chapter, many dentists allow their staff to treatment plan and the dentist then does not want to remove a root canal, core and crown from the important treatment plan and total cost. This practice must stop.

How often should I see the dentist? As is the case with medical visits, the visit times were manufactured by dental insurance companies in order to sell insurance. There is no valid data to suggest you go to the dentist every 6 months. You will have to make the decision yourself.

Dental exams and dental restorations will prolong the structure of most teeth. Some people never have to see a dentist. Some people will lose their teeth at a young age no matter if they go the dentist every 6 months or not.

I see tooth retention as this: If you are going to loose your teeth due to decay from lack of saliva or drug use, going to the dentist will only be for the dentist to extract your teeth.

An anecdotal story is of my mother who had periodontal surgery (gum surgery) on ½ of her mouth when she was in her 30s. She is now 80 and both sides of her are mirror images. She still has pockets on her teeth but she has been on anti-inflammatorys on her own for a long time and I attribute this to her retaining her teeth.

I think scaling and root planning only serve to lessen bleeding of the gums in order to facilitate cosmetic work on your teeth.

For the time and money a person can spend on saving one tooth I think extracting and placing a tooth implant to be the best choice. The problem is that people let things get so far that an implant is not feasible due to too many teeth being lost and the cost of the implants which are not covered by insurances.

So typically a person will allow their teeth to deteriorate while waiting for dental insurance. When they finally get the insurance they need full dentures which most people cannot tolerate in their mouth. If they had used the same money they would have been paying to an insurance company on a yearly basis, to see the dentist and have their teeth maintained, most people would be in real good shape and not require dentures or implants.

Preventive Dentistry

I find this topic fascinating in that my opinion of it has changed drastically. My knowledge has not. What I mean by this is that I was a victim of pop-culture when I first entered the dental profession. I followed what the people who paid me told me to do. I followed the doctrine of 6 month recall exams and prophy (cleaning).

Sure, we had data on things such as, after brushing your teeth or receiving a prophy, less bacteria exists on the tooth surface, but there was no data to translate this into decay prevention. Again, the correct question was not asked.

The only thing in dentistry that is preventive is the advice of your dentist to tell you to injest fluoride while pregnant to protect your child's baby teeth, and for children to ingest fluoride from birth until age 8 to protect his adult teeth from decay. I have not seen any data nor anecdotal stories to suggest otherwise.

Other than decay, most damage to teeth is done from bruxing (clenching or grinding), but I have not seen any conclusive evidence to show that educating a patient about this, or fabricating an appliance for the patient to wear in order to protect the teeth from these grinding forces, will work as a preventive action to prolong the function or existence of your teeth in your mouth. Using appliances in your mouth if you grind, will in most cases rid you of headaches and tooth sensitivity.

Topical fluoride (toothpaste with fluoride, or fluoridated water) has some benefit, but real action only occurs if fluoride is ingested (is systemic) and it becomes part of the tooth as it is developing.

Cosmetic dentistry

I liken cosmetic dentistry to costume jewelry. I am not against cosmetic dentistry as long as the patient understands what it does.

There exists amazing cosmetic dentists in this country. Besides being a dentist they are artists. Cosmetic dentistry can be very costly because these specialists are rare and talented. I am amazed at some of their work and the craftsmen (laboratory technicians) they work with to achieve such works of art on the veneers or crowns.

I have found that a patient can have a lump of tooth colored porcelain in their mouth and not know it does not look like a tooth. So most of what a cosmetic dentist achieves is for his ego. Very few if any patients can appreciate the talent and work needed to make cosmetics look great to another cosmetic dentist.

Bottom line, if you want it and can pay for it, go for it. I only recommend cosmetic dentistry be done on a patient if his existing teeth already have large restorations (fillings) or crowns, so that his teeth are not being drilled on only for cosmetics. This means the teeth were already damaged prior to cosmetic work. But this is a personal decision between you and your dentist.

Chapter Seven

Is There Anything Medicine and Dentistry Has to Offer that is Good?

Yes.

Medicine has a role in emergency procedures. If you break a leg, pass out, are bleeding from an accident, physicians are great, as well as hospitals. And also rehabilitation centers.

It is my argument that we should only have emergency physicians and rehabilitation physicians. For example, going to a doctor for a 6 month checkup will not prevent you from contracting cancer or diabetes, but an emergency room can diagnose you once you do have symptoms and the staff can save your life and treat you until you can be placed in a rehabilitation hospital. The rehabilitation hospital would then give you the proper care, insulin, etc. and you would return there periodically to be sure you are doing the correct thing to prolong your life or reduce pain if that is your goal.

The examination is dead. Forget about it!

Dentistry is the same. If you break a tooth or have a tooth infection (abscess) a dentist can repair the broken tooth or remove an abscessed tooth.

Treating decay (cavities) can prolong the time your tooth is useful and painless. But for some, restoring teeth does not prolong the function of your teeth.

I do not see periodontal work saving your teeth if you suffer from inflammation as inflammation is systemic and not isolated to the gums.

What about insurances?

We should only have medical insurance. Medical insurance is for medical problems, not curiosity checks. This means if something goes wrong we have a backup for money. Just think if auto insurance were called "maintenance" insurance? Do we really want to pay $5000/year to have our tires checked and oil changed? I think not. We have insurance to pay for unexpected emergencies, such as a car collision.

As I write this our country is on the brink of socialism which might make this section obsolete. I will give you my opinion of how some medical and dental insurances should function.

I used to have what I call "catastrophic" medical insurance. It was very low cost and had a $2500/year deductible. That is what insurance should be.

My medical insurance did not pay for me to go to a physician and have blood taken in order to go on a wild goose chase and try and find something wrong.

The political changes in our country have slowly been pushing us into socialism by dumbing us down and some of that is thru the use of the term "health care" or "health insurance".

All medical insurance should be catastrophic only, and it would be if the average person was not full of misinformation. It would only cover us if we were hospitalized or needed long term care.

Dental insurance is useless. There are not catastrophic dental problems that auto insurance would not cover, or medical. It is not an emergency to have a veneer fracture or to have a crown fall off. It does not make financial sense to have dental insurance as you never get back more than you pay into it.

Things such as cancer surgery or fracture surgery on a jaw would be covered under medical insurance.

People will go to a bar or purchase a new sofa, but to pay a couple of hundred dollars to fix their teeth? The people are the problem. They have been manipulated into thinking that they should not have to pay for their teeth, that only insurance companies should, and only the government can make that happen. Soon they will want insurance to buy groceries and clothes.

Chapter Eight

What Do You Want to Die of?

That is really what you are deciding if you happen to contract a major illness. Dr. Nortin Hadler (The Last Well Person) put it best when he said "a person can change what he dies of, but not when he dies". What he was referring to is that physicians claim to "save" a life when they remove a tumor or some organ, when really they just prevented the patient from dying from that ailment. But what is meant by "saving" a life? After all, we all die.

A major problem I have seen with physicians is that they practice as if they are taking an exam in medical school. They are in a competitive mode and the competition is to place a name on a condition before another physician does, out of fear of a law suite. Then, once a condition is named, they set out to treat it until it has no name.

To go a little further with this, I like to use the analogy of a relationship. Many people might say that their close friends or loved ones do not really "know" them. For example, I am a dentist by profession, but I am not a dentist by lifestyle. I consider myself to be a naturalist. I do not use coffee mugs that say "dentist" on them. Fortunately my loved ones do know who I am. But I have heard many a people complain that their loved one does not know them. If a loved one cannot really know you, how can your physician? By that I mean, does he know that you are one like me who wants to live a stress free life and not think of what evils a person can have happen to his body? Or are you the one who follows the heard of sheep and wants the doctor to go on a witch hunt to attempt to find and label anything you might have or will have?

Should a person in their eighties be examined for cancer or have cancer removed or treated? Should a patient in his 80s, who had some skin cancer removed be told to stay out of the sun for the rest of their lives? If we are to believe what the cancer specialists say, that long term exposure to the sun causes skin cancer (it does not) then why should a person who has perhaps a few years to live, not enjoy sitting on a chair at a beach until they do? Where is the logic in this recommendation by the skin specialist? After all, he says it takes a long time for the suns rays to cause cancer. The patient only has 1 year to live. This is another example of the physician treating his wallet, and not the patient.

Physicians and dentists fail to consider the big picture. By this, I mean that the big picture is what matters in life, but the details are needed to come up with the big picture(Naryshkin, Understanding Why).

Taking a Risk and Longevity

That is what life is about. Taking a risk. We take risks with many things in life. We take risks with relationships, occupations, our money. Our constitution was written in order that each individual be permitted to take his own risk. Socialism feeds on the fears of the few who do not want any risk in their lives.

I pole vaulted in high school and college and I pushed my tendons and ligaments to their limits. It was fun and I have no regrets. I have aches and pains as I age, but I would not give up my past for a lifetime free from aches and pains.

It was my choice (my parents allowed me to make that choice)to participate in a risky sport. Some might say being a military pilot is risky. But so is driving a car or living in a country that has millions of people in it, some who like to kill people.

I took risk, although at the time I did not think I was taking a risk, in order to fulfill something in my life. It made my life complete. I enjoyed that animal instinct to compete, and challenge injury. I have no regrets.

We all take risks to some degree. Life is not fun without risk (at least I live by this). I do not want to know what I will die of or when. I attack life and I will accept what it gives me. If I have an injury and I want the pain to stop, or my arm to not fall off, I might decide to go to a physician and ask if he can remedy the situation.

I do not want to know if exploring the Amazon, or piloting a military craft will take time off my life. I do not care. If I die when I am 40 or 100, I will have those life experiences. Time living does not make a better life. And if I were to play the devils advocate and agree that all these exams and diets made a person live longer, to what end? Would these practices give you a longer life while in your 20's? I think most advocates claim they add life onto the end. Do you really want to prolong your end of life? Do you want to spend 2 more years in a wheel chair with a diaper at the expense of not eating foods flavored with salt, or drinking your favorite soft drink every day?

Thinking about what I can avoid in order to assure that I will live as long as possible will make any life not have meaning. That is what preventive medicine attempts to do. That is it's goal.

You might be able to change what you die of, but not when (Hadler, 2004). So does it matter to you? Do you want to spend all your emotional and material energy in an attempt to find out if you have a condition that might kill you, and then to have parts of your body cut out or poisoned, only to die of something else? We cannot cheat death. We can beat death by not having it occupy our every thought by buying into this "preventive" medicine thing.

Most of these political fads (eating certain foods are "healthy") claim to stop you from dying from a heart attack. I think the best thing to die from is a heart attack. It is quick and you fall asleep. Would you rather die in a nursing home with alzheimers, or cancer? What do these low information speakers claim we are getting for denying our taste buds and stomachs the joys of salt, sugar and fat?

Chapter Nine

Conclusion

So, what have you decided? Will you choose to live free of the stress put on you thru pop-culture? Or will you follow the crowd and line up to have your body searched to find an evil that will now ruin your life by filling you with stress and fear?

What does the data show? What is meant by "healthy"? Where is the data that demonstrates that "more" (nutrition or antibiotics) is better?

I do not claim that all is as simple as I have shown. I only want to demonstrate that if a professional is to diagnose and treat you, that a diagnosis should be based on scientific data and not consensus, or fear of legal retribution.

If one chose, one could go to see a witch doctor for medical care, but you would know that this was a witch doctor. Problem with our system is that we are all going to the doctor and the result is that of seeing a witch doctor. Our society has deteriorated over the last century and caused this. It is not only the doctors or dentists. It is what the liberal(progressive) politicians have designed in order that we all depend on the government for our lives.

As a military pilot I was taught the limitations of the aircraft. There was no room for consensus. It was stated plainly and we all lived by it. As a geologist I learned to research what I was exploring and to understand that data rules and to follow the data even if I didn't agree with it.

The problem is not necessarily that physicians are not skilled. The problem is that they are performing perfectly good medical procedures when they are not required. (The last well person).

Most fads are just that (fads) because they are based on what a person said, not what the data showed. Currently there is a move for physicians to admit that diets and supplements do not work, but I do not know how far they are willing to go in order to correct their ill thinking. Still, the only thing that can be said about health is that we know starvation for a period of time will make an organism live longer. There is no data on vitamins or supplements that can claim the same.

Like all citizens of the US, I too am a victim of pop-culture as I search the web for articles and the internet only has what a person types into it. They might not accurately reproduce what is in a written journal, and sometimes it is difficult to know if the article is politically sponsored. But I do my best.

There is no need to visit a physician every 6 or 12 months, or at all, unless you are unable to communicate problems due to a poor mental state. Then your only choice is for a physician to go on a wild goose chase and attempt to find something that might be ailing you.

Most dentists I have known are cowards. They are the ones who when asked a question in class would not raise their hands until they looked around to see who else raised theirs. I assume physicians are the same. Perhaps this is a flaw in the system by which medical and dental students are chosen. They are not leaders, but are instead followers of misinformation as long as there is consensus in the misinformation.

I wrote this book in order to make patients and professionals aware of our deficits and how they negatively affect medical and dental care in the US. I did not write about how to solve the problems as I have no ideas on how to solve them. They are problems caused by cultural changes in our society coupled with arrogance of medical professionals, and I do not like them.

I do expect physicians and dentists to be the leaders in educating our populace on what is data backed science and what is simply a belief.

Politicians are politicians for the sole purpose of being voted into office. Our constitution wanted representatives in office. Our politicians are corrupted and do not represent us any longer. The same with dentists and physicians. They act out of self interest, not yours.

I also found physicians and dentists to hide behind complications. They do not use the Copernican Principal, instead they reinvent the wheel at your expense.

These practitioners also do not have a hunger to learn what is correct. They choose to do what their predecessor did in the past, what pop-culture is now, and to not "rock the boat" as they fear having the spot light on them. I see this parallel in politics as well.

I have had the pleasure to take classes in which the speakers had the same opinions I have written about in this book. These speakers are dentists/physicians who are looked at as outsiders due to their unwillingness to follow pop-culture.

I hope that all dentists who have been violating the known data and following beliefs, are embarrassed by what I have written in this book and see the value in changing how they practice.

My purpose was to not point fingers at specific professionals or associations. I will, however, give my support to one organization's journal which I find to be highly non-political and has peer reviewed data oriented articles. That is the AGD or Academy of General Dentistry.

What the future has to hold I do not know. If we do indeed become socialized I imagine what ever a physician or dentist finds will get them the most money, they will prescribe. When the health care system doesn't yield good results, the socialists will simply state that we need more preventive visits, and sooner in life. And they will continue to blame their political enemies for illness.

About me: I only work in institutions where I can practice using data, and I do not have to convince patients to accept a treatment which will not benefit them, or help them. I refuse to even consider working in a private practice as in order to make a decent living I would have to sell patients treatments and perform unnecessary procedures on them.

As for the physicians and dentists who were offended by this book, think about why you were offended.

New—I said earlier that this was not written as a self help book, however, I would like to leave you one prescription I feel we can all benefit from:

RX: One alchoholic beverage a day, one cigar a week.

Have a happy life.

Bibliography

Hadler M.D., Nortin M. "The Last Well Person" McGill Queens University Press 2004.

Hitchens, Christopher "god is not Great" Hachette Book Group USA, 2007

Grant, Eric J. et al, Radiation unlikely to be responsible for high cancer rates among distal Hiroshima A-bomb survivors, Environmental Health and Preventive Medicine, 2009 July,14(4):247-249

No Benefit to Lowering Blood Pressure in Acute Stroke:Study "Drugs.com" Feb 11,2011.

McDonald, Ralph E., Dentistry for the Child and Adolescent,4th edition, The C.V. Mosby Co., 1983

Naryshkin, Evolution, Beliefs and Your Reality, Author House, 2004.

www.ingramcontent.com/pod-product-compliance
Lightning Source LLC
Chambersburg PA
CBHW020529290526
45786CB00002B/805